Blood Pressure Protocol

Kevin Roche

ISBN: 9781980424796

CONTENTS

INTRODUCTION

Welcome to "Blood Pressure Protocol: The Ultimate Guide to a Healthy Blood Pressure Level"! This book provides readers with a detailed discussion on one of the most popular death culprits in the United State: the excess levels of blood pressure.

As a matter of fact, blood pressure plays the key role in maintaining our body's health and wellness. In addition, high blood pressure is also the cause of multiple other associated diseases, including strokes and heart attacks. However, I have written this book to supply you with the foundation knowledge on how to fight against this lethal condition.

Before digging into the main contents of this book, I must emphasize that if you have already been diagnosed with high blood pressure, then the first thing you should do is consult your doctor for drugs and related issues. Make sure that you discuss anything you are going to do with your doctor to promote better results.

By strictly following the real-life strategies laid out in this book, you will be able to dramatically reduce your blood pressure. Having analyzed the potential harms resulting in hypertension, this book indicates an entire process of how to lower your blood pressure level.

Every chapter of this guidebook is compiled and written based on the real-life case studies and experience from me, as well as other prestigious health specialists all over the world.

Last but not least, do not forget to enjoy your own journey when flipping through the pages of this book. When you finish this book, you will sooner or later realize that paring down your pressure is challenging, yet worth trying. Thank you and good luck!

CHAPTER 1. TWELVE KEY STEPS TO LOWER YOUR BLOOD PRESSURE

1) Maintain a Healthy Weight

The very first piece of pressure-lowering advice that every single doctor tells you to do is to lose weight. Losing some pounds allows you to take a major step in reducing your blood pressure. In fact, physical inactivity, along with obesity, is the main culprit for high blood pressure, as reported by the World Health Organization.

The Positive Relationship between Lower Blood Pressure and Weight Loss

Among all the positive lifestyle changes, weight loss has been proven to be the most forceful. As the recently reported statistics reflect, a five-pound loss in weight can lower your blood pressure to a maximum 5 mm Hg, while a ten-pound loss in weight does even better with a dramatic 10 mm Hg decrease.

High blood pressure is most likely to be found among obese individuals, so losing weight tends to promote lower blood pressure in overweight people. Nevertheless, if your body weight is already at a healthy level, and your high blood pressure is due to the matter of family history, then weight loss is of no importance.

But that does not mean that you should not follow the robust lifestyle tips I'm going to suggest as they can still, to some extent, keep your blood pressure down.

The Ultimate Guide to Weight Loss

The plan introduced within this book sets up an achievable goal for people in nearly every age group. If you insist on strictly following this program in one month, a little safe loss in weight will help you realize how essential it is to lower your blood pressure.

It is highly recommended by health specialists that you should only lose between one to two pounds every week. Not only does this rate let you target the amount of fat loss you're aiming for, you can also maintain a healthy blood pressure.

I have already indicated that just a few pounds of weight loss will help you reduce the mercury millimeters in your blood. But how can you get through this challenging mission without giving up?

Remember that losing weight is a combination of various changes in your diet and daily schedule in your lifestyle. Moreover, the process of reducing weight needs to take time to bring out the best results, so it is critical that you be patient.

Here are ten tips that you should keep in mind to have a decent weight loss procedure.

1. Slow but sure. If you plan to lose some weight, a steady and slow pace is always the top priority. An impatient rate of weight loss might end up bringing up some unexpected extra fat that should have come off.

A proper diet will help you remove up to two pounds (which is equal to one percent of your total weight) per week. Such a safe pace allows you to stay away from health problems resulting from significant weight loss (over three pounds a week).

2. Keep the calories under control. Various scientific studies have proven that the one and only principle is always true, which is to reduce the calories that your body normally consumes no matter how much fat, protein or carbohydrate the diet contains.

3. Have your exercise and eating habits tracked. The majority of surveys on people who try to lose weight found out that those who keep track of the quantity and type of the food they eat tend to be more successful at weight loss.

4. Check your weight at least once a week. Tracking your current weight on a regular basis lets you update your process and keep you on track. In contrast, if you do not follow your weight, it is more likely for you to regain weight unexpectedly. The advice is to use a timer to set up a particular day in the week to check your weight.

5. Mind your serving size. Indeed, portion sizes have been made bigger and bigger in recent years, especially at fast food restaurants. This change also contributes to the overloaded obesity rate of American people.

Particularly, the expansion in size adds more extra calories to your meals, thus making you put on unwanted numbers of pounds. Therefore, eating in smaller bowls or plates is a good recommendation to fool your mind into thinking that you are eating more than you actually do.

6. Reduce the consumption of certain foods, or completely get rid of them. A major change to your dietary habits is to cut down on the amount of foods which are high in calories. For instance, fried dishes include double the calories found in the same foods broiled or baked.

7. Choose calorie-free beverages. Water is always a perfect option, of course, as well as other unsweetened liquids. Also, you should make sure to avoid sugary drinks at all cost as they are extremely terrible choices for satisfying your thirst.

8. Divide your ordinary meals into small and frequent ones. Lots of studies suggest that smaller, yet more frequent meals allow you to lose weight more efficiently. The scientific evidence for this piece of advice is that calories are burnt while your body digests the food.

That is also the reason why many articles and TV shows recommend that you divide your daily diet into five distinct meals. Moreover, eating frequently lets you suppress your hunger and maintain the balance of your blood sugar level.

9. Substitutions. Reducing the original food consumption is undoubtedly much harder than replacing it with more healthy foods. Instead of tormenting yourself about what you can or cannot eat, pay attention to things that you should eat *more of.*

10. Take up exercising as a new habit. In addition to a healthy balanced dietary plan, it is best to combine it with a physical activity program. This is always regarded as the most feasible solution to keep your weight under control, thus promoting better outcomes for your pressure-lowering program.

2) *Pay Attention to Salt Intake*

An ugly truth is that salt, one of the most popular condiments, can become a poisonous element if its consumption surpasses the safe amount. Too much salt included in your daily meals can eventually lead to severe health problems such as stroke, heart attack, and high blood pressure. Therefore, cutting down on salt intake is also an ideal solution to lower your blood pressure.

How Much Salt is Enough?

It is recommended that a maximum amount of 1,500 mg of sodium be taken in every single day. But how does sodium differ from salt? The sodium we are eating daily is mostly stored in salt, so salt can be regarded as the transport means of mineral sodium.

However, remember that high blood pressure also stems from an excess in mineral sodium intake. The National Academy of Sciences has addressed the fact that our bodies only need 500 milligrams of sodium a day to function properly.

In fact, besides using salt as a common seasoning, it is also hidden in lots of processed foods, which tend to be overconsumed. Therefore, if you want to reduce your blood pressure, pay extra attention to foods that contain high amounts of salt.

Pragmatic Salt-Cutting Methods

Salt has long been infamous for increasing humans' blood pressure, and this condition is demonstrated to be directly associated with excess sodium consumption.

This connection was officially confirmed when a study called INTERSALT was carried out. INTERSALT conducted large-scale research on over ten thousand women and men whose ages ranged from 20 to 59 from 52 different global populations.

The study found out that those who consumed below 1,256 mg of sodium on a daily basis were likely to have lower blood pressure. On the other hand, those who ate more than the sodium intake baseline tended to develop higher blood pressure, as well as other heart-related diseases as they grew older.

Next, my book is going to emphasize eight simple, yet potent tips for you to cut down on the amount of salt taken in.

1. Opt for fresh foods. The first change to bring into consideration is to substitute your bad food supply with whole unprocessed and fresh foods. The principle behind this modification is that nearly all unprocessed, natural vegetables and fruits only contain an insignificant amount of sodium.

In addition, try to look for frozen or fresh produce that contains little to no salt listed on the label when you browse the supermarket.

2. Take what is written on food labels into careful consideration. Thus, you will be able to make a quick comparison among different brands. Things you should notice on such labels are baking soda, MSG, and sodium-related components.

If you keep this piece of advice in mind, you will be blown away by the fact that there is a surprising difference in the amount of sodium contained in different products. So, opt for cans, bags, and boxes whose labels read "sodium free" or "low sodium."

3. Adulterate foods which are rich in sodium, and rinse processed foods. To be specific, do not forget to rinse the low-sodium canned foods to squeeze off the remaining salt. Additionally, refrain from adding salt to your dishes when cooking.

4. Get rid of seasoning packets. Try seasoning the dishes by yourself, and reduce the consumption of canned foods as much as possible. Common condiments like ketchup, pickles, olives, and mustard should also be limited to a minimum amount.

5. Remove convenience foods from your diet. To be specific, any type of food that comes along with a bag or box needs to be reduced. Consider making your meals in a quick and convenient way instead of grabbing those unhealthy takeaway fast foods.

Moreover, try to flavor your dishes with salt-free condiments, including seeds and nuts, vinegars, peanut butter and dried fruit, which can be useful in similar situations.

6. Remind the waiters to reduce sodium when eating out. Do not hesitate to make specific customization options to your order, and require your dish to be served without salt. Besides, you can also ask them to prepare dressing and sauces separately without adding to your foods beforehand.

7. Replace salt with spices and herbs. Homemade meals are still the best choices as you are totally clear which ingredients you are adding to your dishes. Instead of salt, try using spices or fresh herbs to season your foods.

For example, such spices and seasonings like cumin, nutmeg, cinnamon, lime juice, wasabi paste; herbs like parsley, chives, basil, cilantro, rosemary are all regarded as perfect alternative options.

8. Say no to salt shakers. Just a small pinch of salt contains approximately 160 mg of sodium, that's why you should be extremely cautious. Avoid using salt by opting for many other available substitutes, including garlic, garlic powder or fresh ginger.

3) Unleash the Hidden Power of Potassium

American people tend to have issues with mineral balance in their bodies. As I have stated in the previous section, high salt intake has long been known for rocketing your blood pressure. In fact, another significant element that we need to mention when discussing about blood pressure is potassium.

Although potassium serves as a stunning mineral for our health, it is not well-known as the love for processed foods has blinded us for too long. Therefore, my book intends to emphasize why it is vital to consume an adequate amount of potassium regularly.

The Benefits of Potassium Consumption to Blood Pressure

The way potassium and sodium interacts with each other plays the dominant role in causing high blood pressure. This segment is going to briefly present how this wholesome mineral can positively impact your blood pressure.

First of all, potassium can place a useful influence on the insides of your arteries. Within these thick blood tubes, the part which is responsible for emitting nitric oxide, a chemical substance that helps sooth your vessels, is the endothelial cells.

A higher amount of potassium consumption allows those cells to multiply the nitric oxide being released. As a result, since your blood vessels are cared for, you will be able to reduce your blood pressure. Higher potassium intake also lets you form potassium channels which function as the cell's gateways.

In addition, a lack of potassium, along with a sodium surplus is the main cause of fluid retention and higher blood pressure in your body. Hence, by making up for the potassium levels you are missing, additional sodium and fluids will be removed via the urine, thus cutting down on the pressure on your arterial walls.

Another reason leading to increasing blood pressure is that your nervous system is triggered by the lack of potassium. Additionally, a potassium shortage also results in the stimulation of the renin-angiotensin system, encouraging the renin production process and causing high blood pressure.

How to Eat More Potassium Daily

Here are ten feasible methods that you can easily apply to take in an appropriate amount of potassium for your body on a daily basis.

1. **Strictly follow the list of these must-have foods that are famous for being rich in potassium:** two kiwis, one package of fresh spinach , one can of low-sodium V8, two cups of nonfat yogurt, one cup of soy milk (homemade milk cocoa is preferred), and one banana. Nevertheless, you can also squeeze the liquid out of all these foods to save time while still keeping the mineral value of them.

2. When eating out, at restaurants in particular, **opt for salt-free baked potatoes and grilled salmon,** which is unseasoned.

3. Choose **salt-free pistachios** when you want to have some snacks.

4. Instead of mayonnaise, **avocado** can also be a good alternative as a spread for sandwiches.

5. **Combine your omelet**, which is suggested to be made of egg whites, **with some fresh spinach**.

6. Try looking for **cantaloupe cubes** which are usually precut at grocery stores.

7. Include **fresh potassium-rich vegetables** in your meals such as red peppers, cauliflower, carrots, white beans, broccoli, tomatoes and so on.

8. **Sandwiches with peanut butter and bananas** are also perfect

choices for potassium consumption.

9. Add **prunes, apricots, and dried figs** to your breakfast dishes.

10. Eat fruits that are rich in potassium like **bananas, kiwis and orang**es whenever you can.

4) Uncover Magnesium's Potentials

In addition to potassium, magnesium is also a vital mineral that helps you decrease your blood pressure dramatically. More details about magnesium and its applications to pressure lowering will be discussed later in this book, but this part focuses on how to have decent magnesium consumption in our daily lives.

Why is Magnesium Highly Appreciated?

According to the famous series of DASH studies, the first solution to blood pressure reduction regarding lifestyle modifications are combining three different minerals; namely, calcium, potassium, and magnesium. However, these types of nutrition are recommended to be taken in the form of foods instead of supplements. This method has been proven to be an effective approach to gradually solve high blood pressure.

When it comes to the suggested amount of magnesium consumed every day, it is nearly 320 mg for woman, while for men it is 429 mg. Nevertheless, the ugly truth is that the majority of American people do not consume magnesium to this required amount. To be specific, only 52% of us succeed in doing this every day.

According to lots of previous scientific research, people who have a diet that is high in magnesium tend to reduce the risk of encountering high blood pressure later in their lives. The most recent study reported that an amount of 486 mg of magnesium each day is enough to fight off high blood pressure, as well its associated problems.

A possible measure to increase magnesium intake is to take supplements, but scientists do not encourage these pills. At least twenty clinical trials have already revealed that magnesium supplements have very little to no positive impact on high blood pressure. Therefore, boosting magnesium intake in the traditional way, although it might take very long, still remains the most potent solution.

How to Insert Magnesium into Your Daily Meals

1. **Drink a cup of coffee every morning.** Coffee and its variants, like espresso, are perfect magnesium options. Moreover, a cup of decaf will be preferred.

2. **Have a hot cup of cocoa before going to bed.** Remember to use soy milk with unsweetened cocoa powder for the best effects.

3. **Cook spinach in fat or oil with some raisins and pine nuts** over heat until they turn completely brown.

4. **Molasses is also an ideal source of magnesium which can be utilized in baking.** Also, you can add this type of seasoning liquid into your coffee or oatmeal.

5. **Go for nuts.** Nuts have always been renowned for their magnesium-rich nature.

6. **Pumpkin seeds which have already been roasted are a superb kind of snack,** as one ounce of pumpkin seeds contain 75 mg of the healthy magnesium. Besides, these seeds can be easily found in any supermarket.

7. **Opt for tofu-related dishes.** ½ cup of tofu is reported to contain 50 mg of magnesium with only 88 calories.

8. **Use Latin flavors instead of conventional ones, and you should replace your side dishes with black beans.** Indeed, they include a significant amount of magnesium.

9. **Add buckwheat pancakes to your Sunday breakfasts.** A simple cup of buckwheat flour contains more than 300 mg of magnesium.

5) Yogurt for the Win

In fact, yogurt has a long and prime history. It was considered as one of the primary food sources in Russia until the beginning of the 1900s. At that time, the frequent yogurt consumption was regarded as the major reason why Bulgarian peasants can live for such an unusually long time.

Although more solid evidence needs to be found in order to prove its lifespan lengthening effects, yogurt is undoubtedly an indispensable solution for lowering high blood pressure. Along with the predigested proteins that assist with nutrition absorption, it also provides healthy bacteria that enhances your immune system.

That brings me to the main focus of this section, which is increasing your calcium consumption, one of the three most essential minerals for lowering blood pressure.

How does Calcium Consumption Help with Blood Pressure Regulation?

As we all know, calcium contains a small element that has a pressure-reducing effect. Nevertheless, high-calcium products are demonstrated to promote a much stronger association with lower blood pressure, so this book is going to emphasize how those connections are formed.

First and foremost, if your diet lacks calcium, a condition called "calcium leak" might happen with your kidneys. Specifically, those who encounter this problem tend to release more calcium through urine, thus messing with the mineral metabolism balance included in the regulation of blood pressure. Hence, decent calcium consumption helps repair that leak as it provides your body with the necessary minerals and lowers your blood pressure as a result.

In addition, dairy products are reported to contain a protein that is derived from milk which can naturally reduce your blood pressure. This type of protein functions as an ACE inhibitor in some ways because it disturbs the angiotensin transformation into an angiotensin type II that is infamous for increasing your blood pressure.

Top Tips for Equipping your Daily Meals with Yogurt

A cup of nonfat yogurt can provide 400 mg or above of calcium, along with many other minerals and vital substances with only a limited number of calories. However, eating plain yogurt might make you feel bored if you have to repeat it day by day. Thus, here are some suggestions for spicing up the original yogurt.

1. Combine it with condiments like dill, parsley or garlic. You can also utilize yogurt as a vegetable dip.

2. Mix yogurt with sugar-free fruit preserves, then use it as a dip for fruits.

3. Pour the yogurt onto your oatmeal, then use fresh berries, flaxseeds and a spoon to mix it completely for a healthy yummy breakfast.

4. Replace water with fat-free yogurt in pancakes and baked dishes. This simple replacement will sooner or later make you realize how nutritious and tasty a meal can transform into with just the addition of yogurt.

5. Make a yogurt pumpkin pie. Add yogurt (an 8-ounce cup should be enough) to a proper amount of plain pumpkin, together with a little bit of pie spice and two Splenda Essentials packets. Mix them carefully, then use some diced walnuts as an intimidating topping.

6) Obtain more Plant Protein

For those who are looking for a credible piece of advice regarding lowering blood pressure in a natural way, plant protein selection always remains the top priority. Particularly, scientists have concluded that adding soy to your dietary plan helps you significantly reduce the obsessive millimeters of mercury.

Soy has gained its reputation for being a rich source of plant protein, providing the important amino acids that any human diet requires. Unlike other types of animal protein, it does not contain cholesterol. Additionally, a suitable amount of soy protein consumption has been proven to cut down on your blood pressure while animal protein does the opposite.

The Greener, The Better

Replacing animal protein with plant protein allows you to have a stunning dietary strategy. Not only will it help you reduce your blood pressure, but it will also let you cut down on the additional pounds on your body. As a matter of fact, vegetarians tend to be leaner than those who are not, not to mention that they are less likely to develop high blood pressure.

A large-scale scientific study that investigated approximately five thousand middle aged people in four different countries discovered people who consumed more vegetable protein instead of animal protein tended to have lower blood pressure.

In Which Way Can Soybeans Reduce Blood Pressure?

The heath-related advantages of soy have long been documented and are put down to various mechanisms such as antioxidants, phytoestrogens, and amino acids. Let's take a closer look at all the possible culprits.

Firstly, an outstanding sign of a well-working artery is the constant production of a relaxation chemical in our blood vessels known as nitric oxide. For those who have high blood pressure, the nitric oxide production is usually compromised. Moreover, the arteries are no longer able to efficiently dilate to respond to the synthesized nitric oxide.

Therefore, the isoflavones included in soybeans have the ability to improve the production of an enzyme which is responsible for producing nitric oxide. As a result, decent soy consumption can relax your arteries, thus easing your blood pressure.

In addition, plant protein is an unlimited source of arginine, a type of amino acid, which is reported to be acutely beneficial for your arteries as it provides a strong foundation for your body to accelerate the nitric oxide production. Besides lowering blood pressure, nitric oxide also plays a key role in preventing blood clot formations within your vessels that could lead to sudden strokes or heart attacks.

What's more, soybeans are also a perfect option for enhancing your kidney's state of health. They are capable of paring down the levels of blood sugar, as well as increasing the sensitivity of muscles to insulin. Consequently, it can protect your body from being resistant to insulin, reducing the chances of you developing hypertension.

How to Supply your Dietary Plan with Soy Protein?

1. **Replace cow milk with soy milk.** Use it whenever you can, for example on cereal, in puddings, in baking, in shakes, as well as anywhere else which you typically use cow milk.

2. **Regularly eat unsalted and steamed edamame.**

3. **Use dry-roasted, unsalted soy nuts as a type of snack.** You can also mix them with your yogurt, or use as an additional crunch by dropping them into your salad. Because soy nuts are very portable, you can keep them in a small bag and bring it along to almost anywhere.

4. **Include more tofu in your daily meals.** Its applications are pretty flexible because it can be easily mixed with many other ingredients. Besides, it can be cooked in numerous ways, including stir-frying, blending for smoothies, or just simply being served as a side dish.

5. **Tempeh is a good choice in addition to tofu.** The difference is that tempeh has a chewier and firmer texture than tofu. Tempeh can also quickly absorb any flavor mixed with it, so it is a great source of plant protein.

6. **A banana sandwich with soy nut butter** is a must for busy people.

The Scientific Secrets behind Dark Chocolate

There is nothing more convincing than letting the figures and statistics speak for themselves. Hence, I will mention a series of large-scale studies based in Germany that aimed to figure out how eating chocolate and lower blood pressure are associated.

According to the research, it is reported that a little bar of chocolate each day can help you significantly reduce the risk of lethal strokes and heart attacks by a whopping 39%. After investigating the dietary habits of twenty thousand middle aged Germans during a whole decade, scientists from the German Institute concluded that those who ate a chocolate bar every day tended to have a much lower blood pressure compared to those who did not.

The question is, why is dark chocolate so powerful?

The fact that eating chocolate can cure hypertension may sound so unbelievable, but there are solid scientific explanations for this nature of this so-called junk food.

Like calcium, chocolate can also be considered as an ACE inhibitor in our body. In case you do not know, there is an enzyme called angiotensin-converting enzyme which is responsible for transmuting angiotensin type I into angiotensin type II. However, angiotensin type II is blamed for constricting your arteries.

Chocolate has been found to emit an anti-ACE effect just like the ingredients included in blood-pressure-reducing prescription medication. A Swedish study discovered that a frequent consumption of chocolate remarkably decreases the level of your blood pressure.

Besides, cocoa contains lots of flavan-3-ols, which is the polyphenol flavonoids' major subclass. By stimulating the nitric oxide production, flavan-3-ols is demonstrated to help widen your arteries. In addition to directly boosting the production of nitric oxide, these flavonoids can also enhance the process of manufacturing and absorbing it.

Obviously, the endothelium's dysfunction is a typical characteristic found in those who develop high blood pressure. Thus, a proper amount of cocoa intake every day is able to reverse this dysfunction, as well as accelerate the blood flow.

Finally, it is widely known that a blood clot can easily lead to a stroke or heart attack as it makes its formation in ruptured plaque, blocking the natural blood flow. When the clot starts taking a toll on your brain and heart cells, a fatal stroke or heart attack can occur at any time. Thus, chocolate intake has been shown to decrease such blood clots in size thanks to the appearance of flavan-3-ols.

6 Simple Tips to Increase the Daily Dark Chocolate Intake

1. A hot cup of homemade steamed chocolate is a good choice before sleep, not to mention that it is also extremely easy to make.

Mix two spoonfuls of sugar-free cocoa powder into a cup, along with soy milk and a little bit of sweetener, then heat it briefly in the microwave. Add some delicious fat-free toppings, and you are done! Such a healthy and attractive beverage, isn't it?

2. Opt for chocolate-associated products which only have one origin. For example, it is reported that Java and Madagascar cacao beans contain twice as much flavan-3-ols as cacao beans in other different areas.

3. Use sugar-free cocoa powder and chocolate squares in baking more often as they both promote an antioxidant effect.

4. Dip a banana into hot chocolate chips, then add some whipped cream as a topping.

5. Drink a cup of tea before going to bed while eating one to two dark chocolate bars.

6. Prepare various squares of dark chocolate and remind yourself to eat them on a daily basis. Due to their portability, you can also bring them along to public places like when you go out on a trip.

7) Wise Red Wine Consumption Does Wonders

Red wine has been shown to reduce the blood pressure if your consumption remains at the moderate level. However, if red wine intake goes over the safe baseline, you can end up increasing your blood pressure as a consequence. Therefore, red wine should only be taken into consideration if you can make sure that you are a responsible drinker.

Uncover Red Wine's Pressure-Lowering Assets

In fact, red wine consists of two natural substances which are believed to make great contributions to preventing hypertension, including ethanol and some polyphenols like procyanidins and resveratrol. Many scientific studies have concluded that ethanol has the ability to fight off circulatory disease by soothing and widening your arteries, thus enhancing the natural blood flow and reducing blood pressure.

Additionally, ethanol is also capable of improving the production of polyphenols during the wine manufacturing process, so your intestines will find it easier to absorb it. To be more specific, polyphenols are regarded as the vital chemical substances that make red wine stand out from other kinds of alcoholic liquids.

Scientifically, polyphenols can be classified into two primary groups, which are *flavonoids* (such as the anthocyanins, or the flavan-3-ols that I have already noted in the dark chocolate segment) and *nonflavonoids* (such as phenolic acids, stilbenes or resveratrol).

There is a wide variety of similar antioxidants contained in grapes, the majority of which are situated in the seeds and skin. Therefore, in order to tap into the huge source of polyphenols, make sure that you choose red wine over white wine.

Whereas white wine is produced by squeezing the juice of the grapes, red wine goes through the fermenting process, with the grapes' seeds and skins being macerated. As a result, red wine can contain up to ten times more polyphenols than the white wine does.

How does Red Wine Lower Blood Pressure?

Here is a summary of how moderate red wine consumption can be overwhelmingly beneficial to your arteries.

I have emphasized multiple times that nitric oxide plays a very essential role in soothing your blood vessels, thus reducing blood pressure and improving your cardiac health. The procyanidins, quercetin and resveratrol included in red wine can significantly boost this nitric oxide production. Remember that high blood pressure patients tend to be lacking in this oxide, so their vessels might get constricted easily.

To be specific, you may wonder which type of red wine is the best for improving vasolidation. According to a scientific study based in Italy, red wine which is produced using wooden barrels, especially oak barrels, have presented better vasolidatory impacts than the wine produced in the conventional way as it consists of more tannic acid and quercetin.

What's more, a little bit of red wine at dinner can enhance the blood sugar regulation, as well as reduce the risk of type 2 diabetes development, leading your blood pressure to decline. A series of fifteen studies in approximately 370,000 people documented that those who kept up with frequent red wine consumption cut down the chance of encountering type 2 diabetes by nearly 30%.

As people who come down with hypertension are likely to have inflammation in their arteries, drinking red wine on a regular basis lets you prevent such inflammation from developing by releasing a chemical substance that reverses the process. In a clinical trial involving 67 Spanish men, they were required to drink 30 grams of red wine, red wine which was dealcoholized, and gin every single day during a four-week period.

Eventually, it was concluded that red wine, which is basically the combination of polyphenols and ethanol, was a perfect choice regarding anti-inflammatory solutions.

Lastly, red wine has been proven to block the growth of bulge, known as the fat cells which are immature. The reason for this benefit was figured out by a group of Korean scientists. Specifically, red wine contains a compound called piceatannol that not only helps you lower your blood pressure, it can also help you lose weight.

8) The Fantastic Four

This chapter has hitherto formed a backbone for a thorough blood-pressure-lowering plan, including a dietary plan which is high in magnesium, potassium and calcium. Whereas the use of nutritional supplements is usually not appreciated, there is some scientific evidence stating that a few specific supplements are totally safe to use.

However, whether taking supplements is a smart move is still in heated debates, so this section should only be regarded as a reference. To put it another way, it is vital that you bring them into consideration before adding them to your pressure-cutting strategies.

Why Supplementation?

As a matter of fact, not everyone can follow a strict perfectly nutritious dietary plan. Besides healthy lifestyle modifications, supplements can be a good choice if we can't obtain enough pressure-lowering ingredients we need.

Although I strongly believe that food consumption remains the best type of nutritional intake, there are times that supplements are truly helpful. Here is The Fantastic Four, which has been scientifically proven to promote outstanding results.

Name of supplement	Recommended prescription
Omega-3 fish oil	1 to 2 grams per day
Vitamin D3	Between 1,000 to 2,000 IU per day
Vegetable juice (low in sodium)	1 cup a day
Coenzyme Q10	Between 100 to 300 mg per day

Let's have a closer look at how each of the above supplements functions in order to maintain the balance of your blood pressure levels.

The Powerful D

How come taking vitamin D is beneficial to your blood pressure? It has been reported that those who develop hypertension tend to have a lower amount of vitamin D than those who do not. A series of clinical trials have also concluded that regular vitamin D consumption leads to a two-milligram decline in blood pressure.

Therefore, now this book is going to provide you with a deep insight into the benefits of vitamin D consumption, along with the role of calcium as its partner.

First and foremost, calcium and vitamin D are regarded as two supplements that get along very well with each other. Vitamin D can enhance the process of absorbing calcium within your body. Besides, it also has the ability to improve your calcium regulation in your blood vessels.

In order help your vessels remain flexible and relaxed, it is important that the amount of vitamin D and calcium intake be balanced. In fact, if your body is not supplied with a decent amount of vitamin D for calcium regulation, the additional calcium will be deposited inside your arterial walls, making them become stiff and hardened.

I have already noted previously in this book that renin is responsible for converting angiotensin type I to angiotensin type II, thus raising your blood pressure. Vitamin D, instead, serves as an ACE inhibitor that suppresses the kidney's renin production.

Coenzyme Q10 – Your Second-Best Friend

The lack of coenzyme Q10 in high blood pressure patients has suggested that this enzyme is directly related to pressure regulation in some ways. Hence, scientists have doubted if supplying CoQ10 can help lower your blood pressure. According to an Australian series of 12 clinical trials that included 362 high blood pressure patients, CoQ10 was proven to enhance their condition dramatically without the occurrence of side effects.

Although its positive effects on hypertension still need to be scrutinized, it is fair to say that coenzyme Q10 is a really safe supplement to use on a regular basis. But how exactly does it help to reduce your blood pressure?

One popular culprit of hypertension is oxidative stress, which is a circumstance that describes how too much marauding – harmful molecules – destroys your endothelium, obstructing the bloodstream's ability to dilate and relax. To protect your body from being attacked by these free radicals, antioxidants are present to stop them from spreading further and causing a chain oxidation reaction, destroying DNA and cells.

Therefore, CoQ10 is a powerful chain-breaking antioxidant that is capable of reversing the artery constriction, thus helping you get rid of oxidative stress and cutting down on your blood pressure levels.

Omega-3: The Ultimate Nutritional Rock Star

The final element of The Fantastic Four we are going to investigate is the fatty acids, which are usually considered as "protective." Fatty acids are divided into two major groups, which are omega-6 acids and omega-3 acids. Moreover, the omega-3 fatty acids are broken down into two more kinds: short-chain and long-chain, both of which are famous for improving humans' health, and more importantly, lowering blood pressure levels.

The same question is repeated, how much omega-3 is enough?

It is scientifically recommended that in order to provide enough nutrients for your heart, you should include at least two meals which are rich in omega-3 every week. Unfortunately, the majority of Americans does not consume to this necessary amount, with about 100 mg taken in per day.

The ideal omega-3 consumption is having fish meals twice a week. Besides eating fish, an omega-3 supplement, or fish oil, is also a perfect alternative choice to reduce your blood pressure. Specifically, fish oil lowers the risk your heart-related problems, as well as promotes a remarkable drop in your blood pressure. Here are some of the major reasons why fish oil is beneficial to your health.

As you grow older, your blood vessels' elasticity starts to decline as the arteries harden. This condition leads to higher blood pressure, and forces your heart to work harder in order to pump enough blood for circulation. Fish oil, in contrast, has the ability to relieve this stiffness.

The second reason why I highly recommend fish oil is that high blood pressure patients tend to encounter endothelial dysfunction, which happens when your endothelium's cells cannot produce enough nitric oxide for your body. It has been suggested that omega-3 fish oil enhances the functions of your endothelium, thereby reducing your blood pressure levels.

You have known that fish oil is able to reduce inflammation in your arterial walls by preventing inflammatory compounds from excessive production when you eat omega-6 fats. What's more, eating fish meals on a daily basis allows you to lose both additional fat and lower blood pressure levels.

9) Reduce Stress

In fact, one of the most terrible impacts of stress on humans' health is accelerated blood pressure. Hence, keeping your stress levels balanced is a key step to putting your blood pressure under control. You might consider yourself as being stress-free, but you may not be able to recognize that the world has changed so much.

In other words, you end up thinking that the amount of stress you are handling is totally normal, and you continue keeping with it until you are tired. However, if you implement these simple stress-lowering techniques, you will sooner or later realize that your mind is gradually getting calmer every single day.

Repetitive Tasks

The first piece of advice to lower your stress levels is to build up a trance-like state within your mind by repeating any activity many times. For example, whispering a specific word over and over again is a good choice, and it is recommended that the word you use describe your desirable state or feeling.

"Peaceful" is one of the most suitable words that can be utilized to help you calm your nerves. After closing your eyes, keep mumbling the word "peaceful" various times until you feel that your mind is actually getting more peaceful, cutting down on the stress you are taking on.

This strategy has been demonstrated to lower your blood pressure as it helps you regulate your breathing while you focus on repeating a word describing peace. Nevertheless, you should make sure that your mind pays full attention to the chosen word without letting it wander near any negative thought, thus lessening the production of stress hormones that accelerates your heart rate.

Music

This may sound familiar, but the type of music that is suggested in this book should have a calming and soothing melody. By listening to such music tracks, you will be capable of reducing your stress levels as it releases a peaceful vibe via meditative sounds. Do it whenever you can, and you will find your life much easier to live.

Retrieve the Good Old Days

Another method of lowering stress levels is to recall your past achievements and successes because they have a magical power to make you feel content and confident in yourself. Moreover, ecstatic memories also allow you to have faith in the moment you are living, thus strengthening your problem-dealing ability.

Write a Thought Diary

A thought diary enables you to note down your genuine feelings on any issue happening in your daily life. In this way, you will soon realize the things that are truly annoying, thus making it easier to find the solutions.

Since it is sometimes difficult for you to share your personal problems with others, keeping a journal allows you to address them in another way. According to a series of studies, writing down your issues on paper helps you feel less burdened immediately.

Be Calm

People who find it easy to keep calm, even in stressful situations, tend to have less chances of developing hypertension as stress hormones cannot mess up their body's functions. If your heartbeat rate remains the necessary balance, your blood pressure is more likely to stay at the normal level.

In order to maximize the potentials of this strategy, you should practice it three 15-minute periods a day.

10) Meditation

Research has shown that meditation is a perfect measure to calm your nerves, as well as lower your blood pressure. Therefore, this segment emphasizes the significant benefits of meditation.

Meditation has long been renowned for its stress-relieving effects, and many health specialists suggest regular meditation as a method of treating this mental problem. In fact, practice meditating does not take much time as you only need a few minutes of your free time for a short duration.

Another tip when you meditate is to look for a place where you can comfortably sit down and nobody can disturb you. Moreover, it is recommended that you set up a schedule in which you feel motivated to fulfill the available tasks.

Here are some detailed guidelines on how to have an efficient session of mediation. First and foremost, put on loose clothing, take off any accessory or jewelry which might obstruct your body's circulation. Place your hands on your lap, and let them stay there for a while.

1. Breathe. Take a slow and deep breath while inhaling using your nose. After holding your breath for a brief moment, exhale slowly using your mouth. Repeat the procedure for one minute or more until you feel that your mind has become more relaxed.

2. Aim for inner peace. Try to close your eyes and let your mind wander to a further place where everything is calming and soothing.

If you are staying in a position where closing your eyes is not possible, you can instead lower them to prevent other things from distracting you.

3. Relax. Let your face muscles loosen up, as well as relax your temple, eyes and forehead. You can close your eyes if that makes you feel easier to focus. Simultaneously, feel your neck muscles, shoulders and back relax. You will soon realize that the stress you have been feeling starts going away.

If your mind is clouded with negative thoughts, consciously try to throw them away by paying attention to an imaginative word or object. If you start to feel much better after a meditation section, open your eyes again and continue doing what you have left hanging.

This tip specializes in quick meditation sessions, but if you have more free time, it is suggested that extensive meditation solutions are implemented so that the benefits are maximized.

4. Longer sessions. An ideal place to meditate is somewhere nobody can bother you. Firstly, focus your attention on your breathing pattern and rhythm as these characteristics tend to become irregular during stressful circumstances. As a consequence, the oxygen provided to your body will be limited, not to mention that the levels of your blood pressure also increase dramatically.

5. Visualize colors. Another effective measure when meditating is to imagine that your breath has a blue color while you are inhaling and exhaling. Likewise, picture the stressful zones within your body are in burning red, so the blue breath can do a quick sooth and calm those red spots until you feel more relaxed.

It is time to turn to your brain, and focus on areas where inflammation exists. Try to avert the flow of calming breath to your brain and slowly let it get out of your mind. Imagine that you open a small door from within your brain that plays the role of a gate where your breath filters out.

Repeat the process over and over again until you are sure that your brain has been well-cleaned, tidying any dislodging memory or clogged area that exists. Finally, you will be able to relieve all the tension built up within your body.

6. Let your mind wander. Allow your mind to rest even more efficiently by picturing yourself in a dream-like location. This can be any destination that you have wanted to visit but never have a chance to do, and do not forget to imagine as many details about the scenario as possible.

For instance, if you want to let your mind travel to the sea, try to figure out what the beach's surface color is. Notice how the tides are moving, or if there are any birds flying on the horizon. Also, pay attention to the color of the clouds so that you truly believe that you are currently at that place.

7. Let go. Do whatever you want to do, ranging from playing with the water to walking by the coast. Listen to the ringing sounds of the waves, along with smelling the salty scent of the air. Look at the clear blue sky and enjoy the sun rays massaging your face.

Additionally, the wind is surrounding you, messing up your hair and blowing your stress away. Picture some details relating to what you wear and the way you look. The sand is gliding among your toes while you are standing still with both arms stretched out.

11) Regular Exercise

There must be a good reason why the majority of health agencies around the world use regular exercise as the core strategy for the treatment of hypertension. In fact, couch potatoes encounter a fifty-percent higher risk of getting high blood pressure.

Moreover, scientists have found out that exercise is one of the best ways of widening your arteries, as well as reversing the raising blood pressure. In the last general solution for cutting down on blood pressure, we will get out of the kitchen and opt for the park, pavements, swimming pool or the gym.

The Natural Blood-Pressure-Reducing Therapy

It is reported that jogging for at least 30 minutes a day promotes the same effects as taking hypertension medicines. Cardio exercise like swimming, biking or walking can reduce your blood pressure by 5 to 10 millimeters of mercury.

As a result, by lowering your blood pressure levels, you will be able to dramatically decline your chances of heart attacks or strokes up to approximately 20%. That is a pretty impressive result! Thus, this session focuses on how to properly exercise to achieve similar successes.

A scientific study published in a prestigious journal has documented a series of 54 clinical trials, involving 2,419 attendants in order to analyze the impact of frequent aerobic exercise on lowering blood pressure. Eventually, they concluded that those who exercise regularly tend to experience a decline in both diastolic and systolic blood pressure of about 1.33 mg Hg.

It is essential to emphasize that exercise has been demonstrated to reduce blood pressure of those who have a typical body weight, thus making it credible to state that exercise promotes a blood-pressure-reducing effect regardless of weight loss.

Another research conducted on over 3,000 participants has shown that exercise actually puts a positive impact on hypertension. When sedentary individuals began taking up exercising such as jogging, cycling, or running for at least three forty-minute sessions every week, their blood pressure levels after four months were found to decrease by 1.16 mm Hg in people with high blood pressure.

Exercise Prescription for Blood Pressure Reduction

So far, you know clearly that exercising on a regular basis is recommended to balance your blood pressure levels. Therefore, what we should do now is break it down into small achievable goals. Keeping up with a plan is the key point, but its sustainability is also an important point that you should take into consideration.

Here is a suggested exercise prescription which has been proven to produce outstanding results for those who develop high blood pressure.

- **Frequency:** every day of the week (if possible)
- **Intensity:** light to moderate
- **Time:** the most ideal duration is half an hour of continuous cardio exercise each day
- **Type:** physical activities that strengthen your endurance, including jogging, swimming, walking, or cycling, combined with one to two strength-training sessions twice a week

Top Tips for Regular Exercise Motivation

First of all, remind yourself to keep exercise as one of the top priorities in your daily life. If you constantly note in your mind that exercise is the best prescription for your high blood pressure condition, and enhancing your state of well-being, you will be able to stick with the plan for a very long time.

Another trick for not giving up is to start slow. A short walk in your neighborhood is an optimum starting point, and then you can gradually increase the intensity of your physical activities.

In addition, you had better create a specific target prior to every exercise session. To be specific, setting up a distance and a detailed itinerary when jogging, cycling or swimming allows you to picture the plan more clearly. Do not forget to put on comfortable clothes and shoes, as well as drink enough water during practice.

If you like to have company, exercising with your dog or a friend will make the task more interesting. You may also bring along your MP3 player so that you can enjoy listening to your favorite songs, thus cutting down on the stress you are handling while exercising. Besides, joining a gym is also a good option, as personal trainers will guide you step by step on how to improve your health properly.

CHAPTER 2. MAGNESIUM – A POTENT PRESSURE-CUTTING WEAPON

1. The Connection between Hypertension and Magnesium

There are solid proofs showing the evident link between magnesium deficiency and high blood pressure patients. A huge number of epidemiologic studies stated that magnesium and blood pressure have an inverse relationship. To be specific, populations with higher magnesium consumption are more likely to have lower blood pressure levels compared to those do not.

What's more, researchers have also found out that those living in locations surrounded by hard water that has high levels of magnesium tend to have lower risk of encountering cardiovascular disease. Another connection between magnesium and hypertension has been pinpointed in dietary studies. Particularly, vegetarians can significantly lower their chances of this health issue as they consume more magnesium than meat eaters.

2. *Hypertension Prevention with Magnesium*

Blood pressure specialists always work towards a permanent prevention treatment for hypertension. In fact, finding out a possible measure to prevent the growth of a specific disease is as important as treating it. Many patients develop cardiovascular disease although their blood pressure is not diagnosed as hypertension (but is still higher than the normal level).

Therefore, preventing your blood pressure from reaching the pre-hypertension level is extremely essential. According to a health journal published in 1997, the severe consequences resulting from hypertension are reported to increase with blood pressure elevations even though the initial levels are normal.

Although the advantages of proactively preventing hypertension are unlimited, we need to pay more attention to the way we can achieve this ambitious goal. It has been suggested that regular exercise, having a healthy dietary plan, lowering salt intake, and increase potassium consumption are all possible solutions.

Besides these above methods, magnesium addition is an indispensable strategy. As a matter of fact, it has been reported that the most significant effect of magnesium might be preventing the early onset of hypertension. If you are diagnosed with high blood pressure, or you just simply want to protect yourself from this condition, taking a daily dose of magnesium is a smart move.

3. Hypertension Treatment Options

The majority of hypertension specialists suggest that the process of treating high blood pressure requires a combination of different measures, including magnesium supplementation. Despite the fact that increasing magnesium intake is not the only necessary method for curing hypertension, it still provides patients with a thorough approach.

It is widely known that there are two major factors constituting high blood pressure, which are genetic culprits, with genes being the dominant element, and environmental causes, including obesity, diet, smoking, etc. In order to identify effective treatments, all of those factors need to be brought under scrutiny.

Moreover, the blood pressure of hypertension patients tends to increase with time, so it is vital that early treatments be applied when our bodies' conditions can still effectively react to non-drug solutions such as magnesium. However, you should note in mind that improvements may happen after a few weeks, but it can also take a pretty long time.

Indeed, the cells within our body find it difficult to absorb magnesium, while calcium intake is processed rather quickly. Hence, cells need to obtain the needed magnesium first until the amount is enough to prohibit the excessive calcium from invading.

This process can last very long as the ability to assimilate magnesium varies from one to another, not to mention that it also depends on the deficiency degrees. In my case, the benefits of magnesium did not show up clearly until three weeks had passed.

On the other hand, some people still need to combine the use of prescription drugs with magnesium with a view to maximizing the blood-pressure-reducing effect. If that is the case, a decent amount of drug intake can be helpful. I personally recommend non-drug methods, but prescription drugs are not harmful if they are used properly, as they can help prevent heart attacks, kidney damages, strokes and so on.

In fact, conventional medical beliefs have shown that normal diseases are mostly assigned prescription drugs. However, prescription drugs are not the only option, especially in the case of hypertension. The dose of the prescription drugs you are using can be lowered if non-drug approaches like magnesium are combined with medications.

Not only does less medication allow you to reduce the risks of getting side effects, but it also enables you to save a considerable amount of money. Overall, magnesium supplementation is essential.

Different Magnesium Supplement Types

Picking a suitable magnesium supplement form is often not an easy task. Typically, your body can only obtain approximately 30% of the core substance contained in magnesium capsules or tablets. Other best-selling items even trigger a much lower magnesium absorption, with only 10%.

The main reason for this difficulty is that minerals such as magnesium are basically rocks whereas our bodies cannot absorb rocks. A possible solution to this issue is magnesium milk, as a laxative, which promotes very positive outcomes.

As a result, the magnesium supplement you select is a very essential choice. The pure form of magnesium cannot be used in any way since atomic magnesium produces electric charges, thus binding with the atoms existing in nature.

Therefore, there is a wide variety of available magnesium supplements, including magnesium oxide, magnesium sulfate, magnesium carbonate, magnesium chloride, etc. Other types of supplements may contain both magnesium and amino acids so that your absorption can increase dramatically.

For those who have difficulty obtaining traditional types of magnesium, magnesium chelate is a good alternative choice, which can be easily found in health food and vitamin stores. You can also look for many alternative magnesium chelate sources on the Internet.

From my personal experience, those encountering vascular problems should use mineral-free magnesium products instead of combination formulas. Even if it is just for extra nutrients, it is suggested that a dose of magnesium should be taken in separately. Other combination products usually include magnesium in a poor quality that is hard for your body to absorb.

If you find magnesium pills or tablets discouraging to take every day, the liquid form might be a better choice, especially magnesium chloride. Although liquid form is pricier than capsules and tablets, they contain easy-to-obtain types of minerals.

After all, I still highly recommend magnesium pills as they are more convenient and less expensive, not to mention that their effects stay longer after being consumed. But if you cannot absorb them properly, liquid magnesium is your solution.

4. Appropriate Magnesium Intake

Since individual reactions to magnesium differ from one person to another, I strongly believe that you should start taking in a lower amount of magnesium compared to the recommended daily intake, then increase it gradually. For instance, you can start with 100 mg of magnesium up to two times a day. After one to two weeks, you can raise the dose to 320 mg per day for women, and 420 mg a day for men.

An important reminder is to hydrate yourself as regularly as possible as your body get rids of excess magnesium via the kidneys. The best way is to use magnesium supplements is during meals because this will enhance absorption.

For those who are diagnosed with medical problems, they might have to consume a larger amount of magnesium than the recommended dose. If that is the case, you should do that under thorough medical supervision. If you belong to the elderly group, encounter kidney problems, or are using drugs relating to blood pressure treatments, then follow a doctor's advice when using magnesium is vital.

If magnesium intake results in loose or gassy stools, stop using it right away and opt for a safer type of magnesium supplement. Like any new thing you have ever taken up, a trial period is always needed to find out what the best choice for you is. Moreover, you should consider using other minerals like calcium in order to maintain the balance of magnesium with other essential substances.

A disadvantage that you are likely to deal with is finding a doctor who has a detailed understanding of magnesium and its applications. That is also one of the main reasons why I wrote this e-book: to provide evidence-based knowledge regarding magnesium. In the next chapter of this book, I am going to introduce some special recipes that can help you obtain more magnesium through delicious dishes.

CHAPTER 3. 42 SIMPLE BLOOD-PRESSURE-REDUCING RECIPES

1) Breakfast Recipes

Chia Oatmeal

1. Ingredients

- ¼ teaspoon of nutmeg
- ¼ teaspoon of ground ginger
- ¼ teaspoon of vanilla extract
- ¼ teaspoon of cinnamon
- ¼ teaspoon of ground cardamom
- 2 tablespoons of shredded coconut
- 2 tablespoons of chia seeds
- 1 cup of almond milk
- 1 cup of oats

2. Instructions

Pour all ingredients into a bowl. Cover the bowl using plastic wrap, then let it get cold in the fridge for at least 8 hours (preferably left overnight).

Homemade Applesauce

1. Ingredients

- ½ teaspoon of ground cinnamon
- ¼ cup of white sugar
- ¾ cup of water
- 4 peeled, cored, chopped apples

2. Instructions

Mix the ingredients together in a large saucepan. Cook them with intermediate to high heat for at least 15 minutes until the apples get tender. Let the apples cool down, then mash them with a fork or potato masher.

Egg Scramble

1. Ingredients

- ¼ cup of cheddar cheese
- Pepper sauce
- Salt and pepper
- Ground cayenne
- 2 chopped tomatoes
- 4 eggs (already beaten)
- ½ cup of chopped spinach
- 2 chopped garlic cloves
- 1 onion
- 1 potato

2. Instructions

Pour water into a small pot, along with a little bit salt, then heat until the water boils. Add the potato, heat it for another 15 minutes until it becomes tenderized. Eliminate the liquid and cut the potato into pieces once it cools down.

Sauté onion and garlic within a skillet with intense heat, then add spinach and cook for about 2 more minutes until it is wilted. After lowering the heat to medium, pour the eggs inside and wait for 2 minutes. Mix in potatoes and tomatoes, along with pepper, cayenne, hot sauce, grated cheese and salt.

Batter Crepes with Beer

1. Ingredients

- 2 tablespoons of butter
- 2 tablespoons of vegetable oil
- Salt
- 1¾ cups of white flour
- 1 cup of milk
- 3 beaten eggs

2. Instructions

Whisk eggs, milk and beer, then pour the mixture into the flour. Add oil and salt, stir the mixture quickly for five minutes. Let the batter stay still for at least 60 minutes. Preheat the skillet with intermediate or immense heat, and brush a little bit butter on the inside.

Pour 1/3 of the mixture into the cooking pan's central area and make sure that the batter is spread out equally. Get rid of excess batter before moving on. Cook crepe for 2 minutes until it gets golden. Flip and cook the opposite side for half a minute.

Egg Muffins with Sausage

1. Ingredients

- Salt and pepper
- 1 teaspoon of garlic powder

- 1 onion
- ½ can of chili peppers
- 12 eggs (already beaten)
- ½ pound of ground sausage

2. Instructions

Preheat the oven to 350°. Grease some cups of muffin lightly. Cook the sausage with intermediate heat until the outsides turn brown. Pour out the liquid. Mix sausage with all ingredients in a big bowl, then divide the mixture into muffin cups. Bake at least 20 minutes.

Granola

1. Ingredients

- 1 cup of dried cranberries
- 1 cup of raisins
- 1½ cups of honey
- 1 cup of canola oil
- 1 cup of sunflower seeds
- 2 cups of shredded coconut
- 1 cup of wheat germ
- 1 cup of sesame seeds
- 1 cup of pecans
- 1 cup of walnuts
- 1 cup of slivered almonds
- 5 cups of rolled oats

2. Instructions

Preheat the oven to 325°. Mix coconut, sesame seeds, walnuts, oats, sunflower seeds, wheat germ, pecans and almonds in a large bowl.

Cook oil and honey with intermediate heat until they are blended. Stir the oat mixture with honey batter until thoroughly mixed.

Place batter on two separate cookie sheets. Back every side for at least 20 minutes. After taking out of the oven, stir it with raisins and cranberries. Repeat the process to break up huge clusters.

Banana Muffins

1. Ingredients

- ¼ teaspoon of salt
- ½ teaspoon of cinnamon
- ½ teaspoon of baking soda
- 1 ½ teaspoons of baking powder
- ¾ cup of white flour
- 1 cup of wheat flour
- 1 teaspoon of vanilla extract
- ¼ cup of canola oil
- 1 cup of wheat bran
- 1 cup of buttermilk
- 1 cup of mashed bananas
- 2/3 cup of brown sugar
- 1/3 cup of chopped of walnuts

2. Instructions

Preheat the oven to 400°, and grease up the muffin cups. Mix eggs and brown sugar together, then add bananas, vanilla, oil, and buttermilk together. Mix cinnamon, baking powder, flours and salt until combined in another different vessel.

Make a divot in the ingredient mixture, then add wet components and chocolate chips (optional) and stir carefully. Spoon muffin tins with batter, then use walnuts as toppings. Bake at least 25 minutes.

Morning Smoothie

1. Ingredients

- 1 tablespoon of Splenda
- ½ cup of tofu and plain yogurt
- 1¼ cup of frozen berries
- 1 banana
- 1¼ cup of orange juice

2. Instructions

Mix all ingredients until the mixture becomes creamy and smooth, and you have a yummy smoothie!

Cinnamon Donuts

1. Ingredients

- 2 teaspoons of vanilla extract
- 2 tablespoons of butter
- 1¼ cup of milk
- 1 beaten egg
- ½ teaspoon of salt

- ½ teaspoon of nutmeg
- 1 teaspoon of cinnamon
- 2 teaspoons of baking powder
- 1½ cups of sugar
- Greasing spray

2. Instructions

Preheat the oven to 350° and spray a few donut pans. Mix nutmeg, baking powder, flour, salt, sugar, and cinnamon together. Stir melted butter, egg and vanilla in a bowl. Pour the wet mixture into other dry ingredients and stir carefully. Then pour the mixture into separate baking pans and bake for 17 minutes.

French Toast

1. Ingredients

- ½ cup of maple syrup
- 8 challah bread slices
- ½ teaspoon of vanilla extract
- ¼ cup of milk
- 4 eggs
- 4 tablespoons of butter
- 2 tablespoons of sugar
- ¼ teaspoon of nutmeg
- 1 teaspoon of ground cinnamon

2. Instructions

Mix nutmeg, cinnamon and sugar together. Melt butter with intense heat, then whisk vanilla, eggs, milk and cinnamon mixture carefully before pouring it into a container. Dip the bread slices into the egg mixture. Fry them until the outsides turn golden brown. Serve with maple syrup.

Power Balls

1. Ingredients

- 2 tablespoons of flaxseeds
- ½ cup of sunflower seeds
- ½ cup of dried cranberries
- ½ cup of chocolate chips
- ½ cup of raw honey
- 1 cup of peanut butter
- 2 cups of rolled oats

2. Instructions

Use the food processor to pulse sunflower seeds, chocolate chips, peanut butter, flaxseeds, cranberries, oats and honey. Cover the mixture with plastic wrap and let it freeze for half an hour. Make medium-size balls using the mixture and put them on the baking sheet.

Fruit Cups

1. Ingredients

- 1/3 cup of lemon juice
- 1 can of orange-pineapple juice
- 6 bananas
- 1 liquid-removed fruit cocktail can
- 2 liquid-removed crushed pineapple cans
- 1 liquid-removed mandarin orange cans
- 4 cups of frozen peaches

2. Instructions

Mix all ingredients in a bowl together. Put the fruit mixture inside separate plastic cups and cover them with plastic wrap. Let them get cold in the fridge. Take them out 45 minutes before serving.

Yogurt Smoothie

1. Ingredients

- Coconut water
- 1 teaspoon of sprigs and mint leaves
- 2 cups of Greek yogurt
- 1 split vanilla bean
- ½ cup of honey
- ½ cup of water

2. Instructions

Mix honey, water and vanilla bean together in a sauce pan with low heat. Allow the vanilla to simmer for at least 7 minutes. Eliminate the vanilla bean and let the mixture cool down. Use a blender to combine a little vanilla honey with mint, coconut water and yogurt. Blend until the texture becomes smooth and pour it into glasses.

Power Bar

1. Ingredients

- 1/8 teaspoon of salt
- ¼ cup of honey
- ½ teaspoon of vanilla extract
- ¼ cup of turbinado sugar
- ¼ cup of almond butter
- 1/3 cup of golden raisins
- 1/3 cup of currants
- 1/3 cup of dried apricots
- 1 cup of whole-grain cereal
- 1 tablespoon of sesame seeds
- 1 tablespoon of flaxseeds
- ¼ cup of slivered almonds
- ¼ cup of sunflower seeds
- 1 cup of old style oats

2. Instructions

Preheat the oven to 350°. Grease a square pan with a cooking spray. Spread out flaxseeds, almonds, sesame seeds, oats and sunflower seeds on a sheet used for baking. Bake for at least 10 minutes. Pour the mixture into a bowl, then add apricots, cereal, raisins, and currants.

Mix vanilla, almond butter, honey sugar and salt in a saucepan over low heat, remember to stir the mixture constantly for about 5 minutes until it starts bubbling. Pour almond butter into dry ingredients and quickly stir it. Press the mixture manually into an even foundation. Let it freeze for 30 minutes before serving.

Orange Smoothie

1. Ingredients

- 1 banana
- ¼ cup of honey
- 1 cup of pineapple chunks
- 1 cup of orange juice
- 1 cup of mini carrots
- 2 cups of Greek yogurt
- 2 cups of peach slices
- 2 cups of mango chunks

2. Instructions

Mix all the ingredients using a blender and switch on the highest speed until the mixture turns smooth and creamy.

Creamy Eggs and Kale

1. Ingredients

- 4 crusty bread slices
- 2 tablespoons of grated Parmesan
- 4 eggs
- ¼ cup of Greek yogurt
- Salt and pepper
- Grated nutmeg
- A pinch of kale
- 2 tablespoons of chopped leeks

- 1 tablespoon of olive oil

2. Instructions

Warm the oil with immediate heat, then add the leeks while lowering the heat to a lower level. Cook for at least 8 minutes until the mixture is softened. After that, add in kale and cook for 2 more minutes. Sprinkle with pepper, nutmeg, yogurt and salt.

Create four indentations with the kale, then pour an egg into each of them. For better flavors, use salt and pepper to season. Cook with immediate heat for another 2 minutes until the egg whites become firmer. Serve on dishes using parmesan cheese as topping with toasted bread.

2) Lunch Recipes

Scallion Salad and Sweet Potato

1. Ingredients

- ¼ cup of fresh parsley
- Salt and pepper
- 1 teaspoon of honey
- 1 tablespoon of balsamic vinegar
- 2 tablespoons of apple cider vinegar
- 2 tablespoons of Dijon mustard
- 2/3 cup of olive oil
- 8 scallions
- 4 sweet potatoes

2. Instructions

Preheat the oven to 375°. Bake the potatoes for about 45 minutes until they are softened. Let them cool down before splitting them into huge chunks. Continue to preheat a grill at a high temperature. Brush the scallions and potatoes with 1/3 cup of olive oil.

Grill them until they turn tender for about 5 minutes. After that, take them off the grill and split the scallions into small pieces. Mix the olive oil with honey, vinegar, and mustard, sprinkling some salt and pepper. Add parsley, scallions and potatoes to this mixture, then toss it gently until it is perfectly coated.

Couscous Tabouli

1. Ingredients

- 3 scallions
- 2 diced tomatoes
- 2 tablespoons of chopped mint
- ½ cup of chopped cilantro
- 1 cup of chopped parsley
- 3 tablespoons of olive oil
- 1 lemon
- Salt and pepper
- 1 cup of Israeli couscous

2. Instructions

Heat water in a pot with immediate heat, along with a little bit salt and wait until it boils. Add the couscous, then cook until it is al dente for at least 7 minutes. Eliminate the couscous liquid and let it cool down. Mix the lemon juice together with olive oil in order to make vinaigrette.

Sprinkle salt and pepper (optional) for seasoning. Mix the couscous with tomatoes, cilantro, scallions, mint, and parsley until it is thoroughly mixed. Toss the mixture repeatedly with vinaigrette. Allow the mixture to stay still for half an hour before using.

Frittata with Tomato, Fontina and Asparagus

1. Ingredients

- 3 ounces of Fontina
- Salt
- 1 diced tomato
- 12 ounces of asparagus
- 1 tablespoon of olive oil
- ¼ teaspoon of pepper
- ½ teaspoon of salt
- 2 tablespoons of whipping cream
- 6 eggs

2. Instructions

Preheat the broiler, then warm up the butter with immediate heat in a skillet. Add asparagus and sauté for at least 2 minutes. Increase the heat while adding the mixture of egg into asparagus. Lower the heat after adding cheese, then place the skillet inside the broiler. Let it on for 5 more minutes before serving.

Un-fried Chicken

1. Ingredients

- 1¼ cup of cornflake crumbs
- Lemon juice and zest
- 2 egg whites
- ½ teaspoon of hot sauce

- ¼ cup of buttermilk
- ½ teaspoon of chicken seasoning
- 8 chicken thighs
- Cooking spray

2. Instructions

Preheat the oven to 375°, then put a pan on immediate heat. Sprinkle the chicken thighs with seasoning. Mix egg whites, hot sauce, buttermilk and lemon zest/juice in a huge bowl. Use another bowl to add cornflake crumbs, then dip the chicken into this bowl. Manually press them in a gentle way so that the chicken can absorb them.

Put the chicken within the skillet, wait for at least 45 minutes until the skin turns golden.

Paprika Casserole

1. Ingredients

- 6 tablespoons of sour cream
- 2 tablespoons of flat-leaf parsley
- 3 cups of brown rice
- 2 cups chicken broth
- 2 tablespoons of tomato paste
- 1 teaspoon of hot paprika or ¼ teaspoon of cayenne pepper
- 1 tablespoon of Hungarian paprika
- 2 red bell peppers (chopped)
- 2 chopped onions
- 5 chopped garlic cloves
- 1 teaspoon of olive oil
- Salt and pepper

- 2-pound chicken thighs

2. Instructions

Preheat the oven to 350°. Put the chicken in a baking dish, then sprinkle some salt and pepper on top. Bake for at least 30 minutes until thoroughly cooked. In a different saucepan, heat up oil with ¼ teaspoon of salt, onion, garlic, and bell peppers. Cook for 15 minutes, carefully stir until the vegetables get tender.

Pour the hot and sweet paprika into the mixture, then leave it on the stove for 1 more minute. Add the tomato paste and cook for an extra minute. After that, pour chicken broth, along with 2 water cups into the pan. Let the mixture simmer for about 5 minutes so that it becomes thickened.

Place the chicken on a big plate, lay the rice evenly on a dish's bottom, then put the chicken with all juices above. Put the casserole in the oven and bake for 40 minutes. Use a pinch of parsley for toppings.

Chicken Patties

1. Ingredients

- ¼ cup of fresh cilantro
- 1½ cups of diced pineapple
- 1 cup of frozen peas
- 1 cup of white rice
- ¼ teaspoon of turmeric
- 1 chopped red onion
- 2½ tablespoons of vegetable oil
- Salt and pepper

- ½ teaspoon of ground allspice
- 2 minced garlic cloves
- 2 jalapeño peppers
- 1¼ pounds of ground chicken

2. Instructions

Mix the chicken, one garlic, one jalapeño, salt, pepper and allspice altogether. After that, make four patties with the size of ½." Lay the patties on a dish, then put it within the refrigerator. Warm up vegetable oil in a big skillet with intermediate heat, then pour in one onion, along with the remaining garlic, turmeric and jalapeño. Cook for one minute.

After adding salt, water and rice, cook the mixture until the boiling point, then lower the heat to minimum. Let it simmer for at least 15 minutes. Next, you can add the peas, then set the dish aside.

Warm up oil in another skillet with intermediate warmth. Pour the patties into the skillet, cook for about 4 minutes on every side. Toss red jalapeño, the remaining onion, vegetable oil with pineapple cilantro in a bowl. Season with salt and pepper if you want. This dish is served with pineapple salsa and patties.

Pasta Salad

1. Ingredients

- 1 zucchini
- 2 tablespoons of fresh dill or chives
- 1 corn ear
- 2 cups of grape tomatoes or cherry
- Salt and pepper

- ¾ teaspoon of dry mustard
- 1½ teaspoon of sugar
- 1½ tablespoon of cider vinegar
- 3 tablespoons of sour cream
- ½ cup of mayo
- ¼ part of a red onion
- 8 ounces of dry cavatappi

2. Instructions

Boil salted water in a big pot, then add the cavatappi in. Eliminate the liquid and rinse with cold water. While cooking the cavatappi, let the onion soak in cold water for about 5 minutes, then remove the liquid. Whisk pepper, liquidated onion, sugar, vinegar, may, sour cream, salt, oil and mustard in a bowl.

Add the corn, tomatoes, dill, and zucchini into the mixture. After that, cook the cavatappi alongside with the dressing. Make sure to stir carefully until it is perfectly coated.

Stir-Fried Chicken Peanut

1. Ingredients

- ¼ cup of salted peanuts
- 1 Napa cabbage head
- 1 jalapeño pepper
- A little bit of scallions
- 1 ginger
- 2 tablespoons of vegetable oil
- 1 pound of chicken breasts
- 1 tablespoon and 1 teaspoon of rice vinegar
- 1 tablespoon and 2 teaspoons of cornstarch

- 3 teaspoons of soy sauce
- 1 cup of basmati rice

2. Instructions

Firstly, the rice needs to be cooked. While cooking the rice, whisk 2 spoonfuls of soy sauce, rice vinegar with 1 teaspoon of cornstarch. Dip the chicken it and let the mixture thoroughly coat its outsides. Mix 1/3 water cup, 1 teaspoon of rice vinegar or soy sauce, brown sugar and the remaining cornstarch together in a different bowl.

Heat up half of the peanut oil in a big skillet with intense heat. Pour the chicken in and stir-fry it for up to 3 minutes. Put the chicken on a clean bowl, then clean the pan and heat it up again with the remaining peanut oil. When it begins smoking, add scallion whites, ginger and jalapeño for about 45 seconds.

After adding the cabbage, stir-fry the mixture for five more minutes until it turns crispy, then mix the brown sugar and chicken in. Continue stir-frying the sauce for 1 to 2 more minutes. Serve with rice.

Kale with Turkey Rice

1. Ingredients

- 2½ cups of cooked brown or white rice
- Chopped kale
- ½ pound of skinned potatoes
- 1 teaspoon of ground cumin
- 2 chopped garlic cloves
- 1 chopped onion
- 1 pound of ground turkey

- 1 tablespoon of vegetable oil
- Salt
- 3 tablespoons of sliced almonds
- 1 jalapeño pepper
- A little bit cilantro

2. Instructions

Puree ½ water cup, almonds, jalapeño, ¼ teaspoon of salt, and 3 tablespoons of cilantro within a blender until the texture becomes smoother. Warm up vegetable oil in a big pot over intermediate heat, then add ½ teaspoon of salt and turkey. Cook for another 4 minutes while stirring carefully.

When the chicken gets browned, add garlic, onion, and cumin. Continue stirring until softened. Pour in the pureed mixture, kale, potatoes and 1½ water cups. After the water boils, lower the heat to medium level. Let it simmer for about 15 minutes, then serve with rice.

Pancetta Escarole

1. Ingredients

- 3 tablespoons of diced pancetta
- 2 tablespoons of olive oil
- 4 cloves of garlic
- 1 chopped escarole head

2. Instructions

Cool the pancetta so that it turns crispy, eliminate the liquid using a towel. Cook garlic cloves and olive oil in a skillet for about 1 minute. After that, add escarole in and leave the stove on for 5 more minutes.

Use a serving dish to put the escarole and pancetta in.

3) Dinner Recipes

Baked Salmon

1. Ingredients

- 12 ounces of salmon fillets
- Black pepper
- Coarse salt
- Parsley salad with almonds
- Baked squash

2. Instructions

Preheat the oven to 450°. Sprinkle salt and pepper to the salmon fillets, then place them evenly on a baking sheet. Bake 12 to 15 minutes. Serve with the parsley salad and almonds.

Pork Tenderloin

1. Ingredients

- 1 teaspoon minced garlic
- 1 tablespoon of olive oil
- 1¼-pound pork tenderloin
- Salt
- 1 teaspoon of dried thyme
- 1 teaspoon of ground cumin
- 1 teaspoon of ground coriander
- 1 teaspoon of garlic powder

- 1 teaspoon of dried oregano

2. Instructions

Preheat the oven to 450°. Mix the dry ingredients altogether to create the rub, then sprinkle it over the tenderloin. Warm up the olive oil over intermediate heat. Sauté the garlic for about a minute while constantly stirring. After that, put the tenderloin within the pan and cook for another 10 minutes each side.

Use a roasting pan to bake your meat. Finally, cut it into small pieces and enjoy!

Pork Tenderloin with Mushroom

1. Ingredients

- ½ teaspoon of lemon zest
- 2 tenderloins
- ½ cup of fresh parsley
- 1 tablespoon of breadcrumbs
- 1 garlic clove
- Salt and pepper
- 8-ounce cremini mushrooms
- 4 chopped bacon slices
- 5 tablespoons of olive oil

2. Instructions

Heat up 2 tablespoons of olive oil with intermediate heat, then add in the bacon and cook for 8 more minutes. Pour in ½ teaspoon of salt, pepper and mushrooms. Then add garlic and leave it on for an extra minute. Rinse off the meat, then dry it graciously. Cut the tenderloin into even pieces.

Use plastic wrap to cover the pork, then use a meat hammer to beat it until it reaches the thickness of ½." Spread the mixture of mushrooms on those tenderloins, as well as use toothpicks to stabilize the seams.

Preheat the grill with intermediate heat, the use olive oils for grate brushing. Also, brush the pork rolls using oil, salt and pepper. Grill the tenderloins, make sure that you regularly turn the sides until the thermometer reaches 140°. Let it cool down for at least 10 minutes and serve with parsley oil.

Lemon-Onion Chicken

1. Ingredients

- 4 halves of chicken breast
- 9 ounces of spinach
- 2-lemon juice
- 1 cup of chicken broth
- ¼ cup of white wine
- Some thyme leaves
- 1 sliced onion
- ¼ cup of all-purpose flour
- 3 tablespoons of olive oil
- Salt and pepper
- 1 teaspoon of dried thyme

2. Instructions

Season the chicken with pepper, salt and thyme. Heat up olive oil with intermediate heat using a big sauté pan. Pour the flour in a dish, and dredge chicken into batches.

Put the chicken within the pan, sauté both sides for at least 3 minutes each. Then transfer it to the plate and cover it with foil. Combine lemon juice, wine and chicken broth in a bowl and heat it up over intense heat. Cook for at least 10 minutes, then put the pan aside and add in 1½ tablespoons of butter, salt and pepper.

In a microwave-friendly bowl, pour in 3 tablespoons of water and spinach, turn on and leave it for at least 5 minutes. Eliminate the liquid and toss using lemon juice and the remaining butter. This dish is served with the sauce on top.

London Broil

1. Ingredients

- 2 tablespoons of olive oil
- 2 pounds of London broil
- Special Dave's rub

2. Instructions

Rub the London broil along with olive oil. Let it stay still for up to 15 minutes at normal temperature. Heat up a grill pan over intermediate warmth. Put the meat on the pan, grill about 5 minutes each side, then take it down and let it cool down for 6-7 minutes before slicing.

Tuna Steaks

1. Ingredients

- Salt and pepper

- Two tuna steaks (1 pound each)
- 3 tablespoons of olive oil
- 3 scallions
- 3 sprigs of rosemary
- 6 sprigs of thyme

2. Instructions

Chop the thyme, rosemary and scallions and place them within a bowl, along with a tablespoon of oil. Use another dish to season the steaks with salt and pepper. Rub both sides with herb mixture. Cover and let it freeze for 1 to 4 hours.

Warm up the leftover olive oil over high heat. Sear the tuna in a skillet for another 2 or 3 minutes per side. Slice the steaks and you're done!

Coffee Steak with Onions and Peppers

1. Ingredients

- Juice from half a lime and lime wedges
- 1 bell pepper
- Black pepper
- 1 onion
- 2 teaspoons of vegetable oil
- One skirt steak
- Salt
- 1/8 teaspoon of ground cinnamon
- ½ teaspoon of chili powder
- 1 teaspoon of mustard powder
- 1 teaspoon of cocoa powder
- 1 tablespoon of instant coffee

- 2 tablespoons and 1 teaspoon of brown sugar

2. Instructions

Mix cinnamon, mustard powder, instant coffee, 2 tablespoons of brown sugar, 1 teaspoon of salt, cocoa powder, and chili powder altogether. Sprinkle salt and coffee-spice for seasoning. Warm up the vegetable oil over intermediate heat using a medium-size skillet. Sear steak for 3 to 6 minutes per side.

Put the meat on the cutting board, remember to reserve the remaining juices. Add in onion and the leftover brown sugar, along with a little bit salt and pepper. Cook with immense heat for about 5 minutes. After that, pour ¼ water cup and bell peppers into the pan and continue cooking for another 5 minutes.

Stir the mixture with lime juice, you can add more salt and pepper if needed. The steak is served with cornbread and lime wedges.

4) Special Magnesium-Rich Recipes

Tomato Gratin

1. Ingredients

- 2 grape tomato pints
- 4 cloves of garlic
- ¼ cup of olive oil
- 2 teaspoons of fresh thyme
- ½ cup of parmesan
- ½ cup of breadcrumbs

2. Instructions

Cook smashed garlic cloves, thyme, and ¼ olive oil cup with grape tomatoes for about 8 minutes. Mix breadcrumbs, parmesan and the leftover olive oil together in another bowl. Sprinkle the parmesan mixture on tomatoes. Broil for another 3 minutes until the dish turns brown.

Chili Butter with Potatoes

1. Ingredients

- 1 pound of potatoes
- ½ teaspoon of chili powder
- 3 tablespoons of butter
- Salt and pepper

2. Instructions

Add potatoes to salted water in a cold pot. Heat it up to the boiling point, leave it on for an extra 15 to 20 minutes until the potatoes get tender. Eliminate the liquid. Use a pan to melt butter, then add chili powder, along with salt and pepper for seasoning.

Herbal Summer Squash

1. Ingredients

- ¼ cup of fresh chives
- 1 garlic clove
- 2 teaspoons of fresh rosemary and sage
- Salt and pepper
- 1½ teaspoon of white wine vinegar
- 1 onion
- 1 jalapeño
- 3 diced green or yellow summer squash
- 1½ tablespoons of olive oil

2. Instructions

Heat up the oil with intermediate warmth. Add in salt, onions, squash, pepper, vinegar, and jalapeño, stirring until thoroughly mixed. Cover the mixture and leave it on the stove for an extra 6 minutes until the squash turns brown. Remove the lid, then continue cooking for 6 more minutes.

Add in garlic, sage, and chives, then season with salt and pepper for as much as you want.

Cucumber and Watermelon Smoothie

1. Ingredients

- 2 cups of seedless watermelon
- Half-a-lime juice
- 1 tablespoon of honey
- 3 tablespoons of buttermilk
- 2" piece of English cucumber

2. Instructions

Blend lime juice, cucumber, buttermilk and honey using a blender until the mixture turns smooth. Add the watermelon, continue blending until thoroughly mixed. Pour in 1 to 2 water tablespoons so that it reaches the consistency you are looking forward to.

Vanilla Almonds

1. Ingredients

- ½ teaspoon of ground cinnamon
- ¼ teaspoon of salt
- ¾ cup of sugar
- 4 cups of whole almonds
- 1 teaspoon of vanilla extract
- 1 egg white (beaten)

2. Instructions

Preheat the oven to 300°. Mix vanilla extract with egg white, then add in almonds and constantly stir for even coatings. After combining sugar, salt and cinnamon, add egg white to the mixture and continue stirring. Pour the final mixture onto a baking sheet, and bake for 20 minutes. Let it cool down and have a bite!

Cauliflower Rice

1. Ingredients

- Juice of half a lemon
- 2 tablespoons of parsley leaves (chopped)
- Salt
- 1 diced onion
- 3 tablespoons of olive oil
- A cauliflower head

2. Instructions

Trim the cauliflower florets, make sure that you cut off all the stem. After that, break the florets up and pulse for 3 separate batches using a food processor until the mixture looks the same as the couscous.

Heat up oil over intermediate warmth. As soon as it begins smoking, add in onions and constantly stir for even coatings. Cook for at least 8 minutes until the mixture has a golden-brown color. Next, add cauliflower, 1 teaspoon of salt, and cook for 3 to 5 more minutes. Serve in large bowl with lemon juice, parsley, salt and pepper.

Kale Chips

1. Ingredients

- Salt
- 1 teaspoon of za'atar spice
- 1 teaspoon of Mexican oregano
- Olive oil
- 10 dried kale leaves

2. Instructions

Preheat the oven to 225°. Pour kale leaves into a medium-size bowl, pour in olive oil until they become glistening. Sprinkle za'atar and oregano on top, then toss the mixture gently. After that, bake the kale for about 45 minutes to 1 hour. Let it cool down before serving.

Corn Salad

1. Ingredients

- ½ cup of basil leaves
- ½ teaspoon of black pepper
- ½ teaspoon of salt
- 3 tablespoons of olive oil
- 3 tablespoons of cider vinegar
- ½ cup of red onion
- 5 shucked corn ears

2. Instructions

Heat up a pot of salted water to the boiling point, then cook the corn for another 3 minutes to reduce starchiness. Eliminate the liquid. Then pour into cold water for a yellow and bright color. After the corn is cooled down, cut the kernels off the cob.

Put kernels into salt, vinegar, olive oil, salt, onions and pepper in a large bowl. Combine the mixture with fresh basil before eating.

Garlic Cauliflower

1. Ingredients

- Chopped rosemary
- Ground pepper
- 1 chopped garlic clove
- 1 tablespoon of Greek yogurt
- 1 tablespoon of olive oil
- 2 tablespoons of Parmesan cheese
- ¼ cup of chicken stock
- Salt
- 1 chopped cauliflower head

2. Instructions

Boil water in a large pot, then pour in salt with chopped cauliflower for ten 10 minutes. Wait until the liquid is removed, and dry with a towel. Put hot cauliflower with garlic, olive oil, cheese, chicken stock, and yogurt within a food processor. Add a little bit salt and pepper if needed, then pour the mixture into chopped rosemary before serving.

CHAPTER 4. HIBISCUS TEA – THE NATURAL PRESSURE-LOWERING BEVERAGE

1) Why Hibiscus Tea?

According to many scientific studies, hibiscus tea has been reported to significantly reduce hypertension the same way prescription drugs do. However, you may wonder why you should use hibiscus tea if the drugs are just as effective?

First and foremost, hibiscus has gained its reputation for being widely consumed as a lemony drink which is ruby-colored, not to mention that it has been proven to be safer than other hypertension drugs since it does not lead to any side effect.

Despite the fact that hibiscus has been applied in medicine for a while, it is the combination with herbal tea that made it become a top solution to high blood pressure. For example, an amount of 3 cups of tea a day can dramatically reduce your blood pressure levels.

So, how come hibiscus tea can be such a strong weapon against hypertension? Here are some of the most trustworthy explanations from hibiscus specialists:

1. It is suggested that the herb consists of anti-hypertensive and cardio-protective substances which are able to aid the process of

hypertension treatment, as well as other heart-related conditions.

2. Tea promotes an anti-inflammatory effect, which makes great contributions to bringing down your blood pressure.

3. Hibiscus tea contains stunning diuretic properties enhancing the urination frequency, thus cutting down on your blood pressure.

Therefore, after making clear how hibiscus tea can assist the treatment of hypertension, you may feel curious about how much should you drink in order to maximize its potentials? The answer is a spoonful of hibiscus flowers. Using it in boiling water after letting it cool down is an ideal choice.

2) Simple yet Strategic Methods of Consuming Hibiscus Tea

1. If your garden already has a hibiscus plant, here is a simple recipe to make healthful tea from its flowers.

Ingredients

- Boiling water
- Ice
- Lime or lemon juice
- Sugar
- Hibiscus flowers (organic and pesticide-free)
- Heatproof mugs or glasses, jug or teapot

Instructions

After separating the stamens from every flower, use a mug or glass to put the flower in, then cover it with the prepared boiling water. Let the water soak the flower, stir until the water has a blackish purple color.

Next, squeeze a lime or lemon wedge's juice into a glass. You should make sure that the color is bright pink. Put it aside for a while before adding ice.

2. This is another alternative recipe (serving 6 people) for hibiscus tea.

Ingredients

- 1 tablespoon of freshly squeezed lime juice
- ¾ cup of honey, granulated sugar or stevia
- ¾ cup of dried hibiscus flowers
- ¾ inch of grated fresh ginger
- 6 cups of water

Instructions

Mix water and ginger together in a big pot, then boil the liquid over intense heat before turning off the stove. Add sweetener, then stir until the mixture of hibiscus flowers become fully dissolved. Let it cool down for about 10 minutes.

After that, strain the tea into a large heatproof pot or bowl and add lime juice. Keep the pot within the fridge until you want to serve. If you do not have enough time for daily hibiscus tea preparation, you can opt for a type of supplement that contains hibiscus flower extract, including Green Tea Elixir.

3. However, it is not always easy for you to collect real hibiscus flowers. Therefore, you can use this method to make tea from dried hibiscus flowers.

Instructions

Look for dried calyxes from any Latin or Caribbean grocery herb store. Based on your personal taste, the number of dried calyxes added to each cup of water may vary from 1 to 5 teaspoons. After that, use a cup of boiling water to pour the hibiscus powder in.

In order to season and get rid of the annoying taste, fresh ginger slices, sweeteners and cinnamon sticks can be added. Let the mixture cool down for about 10 minutes before taking a small taste to see whether there is enough sweetener or not.

To maximize the power of hibiscus team, a dose of 3 cups a day is an ideal intake to fight off hypertension. If you do not have to use any other medication, a 7-point drop in systolic pressure can be expected within 6 weeks.

Hibiscus tea is able to provide your body with essential antioxidants like anthocyanins which strengthens your blood vessels. As a result, it is capable of preventing your bloodstream from getting narrower, thus reducing the risk of hypertension. As I have stated, a decrease of 7 points is totally believable.

Although this change might not seem important at first, the long-term effect it has on your blood pressure is vital, including lower chances of strokes and heart attacks. Therefore, it has been concluded that the results hibiscus tea promotes is no different than what drugs can do.

3) Top Tips for Using Hibiscus Tea

It is highly recommended that you buy a blood pressure monitor in order to keep track of your pressure levels after using hibiscus tea for a while, thus noticing if it actually helps. Moreover, if you are currently taking prescription drugs, remember to consult your personal doctor before taking up drinking hibiscus tea.

In addition, the ideal hibiscus consumption relies on your age, body weight, and health status. Hence, healthcare specialists will the best choice in terms of finding out how much tea is enough for your own conditions. On average, the suggested daily intake is approximately 10 grams of dry calyxes, or 9.5 grams of anthocyanin.

Generally, the recommended anthocyanin consumption is about 250 mg every four weeks. Another thing that you need to keep in mind is that if you come down with allergic symptoms after using hibiscus tea, stop drinking it and find your doctor right away.

What's more, since hibiscus tea is a rich source of copper, iron and manganese, excess consumption might lead to adverse reactions. Furthermore, because hibiscus tea is applied to hypertension patients, those who have low blood pressures mustn't drink this kind of tea as you may suffer from faintness, brain damage and dizziness. Besides, pregnant women should stay away from hibiscus tea as well.

CONCLUSION

Congratulations on completing the whole "Blood Pressure Protocol: The Ultimate Guide to a Healthy Blood Pressure Level"! Hopefully, the chapters of this book have shed light on what you have been craving to know in terms of credible methods to treat hypertension.

Having made it to the end of this book, I strongly believe that this book has been an informative source for you to rely on when looking for tools that aid the process of lowering your blood pressure. So, what are you waiting for? It is about time you turned the theories into reality.

Make sure that you go through each chapter again more carefully, then practice any strategy that the book suggests. Not until you finish all of them will you recognize how incredible the results are likely to your blood pressure condition. Thank you and I'm looking forward to hearing good news from you!

Thank you!

I hope you enjoyed reading my book!

Finally, if you enjoyed this book, write me an honest review about the book – I truly value your opinion and thoughts and I will incorporate them into my next book.

ABOUT THE AUTHOR

My name is Kevin Roche, and I am happy to announce that I am the author of "Blood Pressure Protocol: The Ultimate Guide to a Healthy Blood Pressure Level". First of all, I want to make clear that I am totally not a health specialist, and I am also not an expert in any related field, nor even have a university degree in it.

So, you must wonder why I can write an entire a guidebook on lowering blood pressure when I am not even a doctor. It all started five years ago when I was diagnosed with hypertension in a cold December. I was a single mom with three children, not to mention that my house is located 200 miles from the nearest medical station.

In short, my budget was not enough to keep up with the medical prescription the doctor had advised. Consequently, I began looking for more natural ways of treating high blood pressure. I ended up finding out that adjusting my lifestyle in an appropriate way allows me to improve my condition without having to take drugs.

Basically, I applied every method which was scientifically backed up by medical evidence, including lifestyle modifications, increasing nutrient consumption, and cooking pressure-friendly recipes. So far, after having a few appointments with my doctor, he has stated that my blood pressure level has now reached the normal level.

Therefore, I have compiled what I have been looking for in the last five years, along with my personal experience and case in this "Blood Pressure Protocol: The Ultimate Guide to a Healthy Blood Pressure Level". I hope my book will help you achieve positive outcomes like I did.

85226698R00069

Made in the USA
Lexington, KY
29 March 2018